# Wishing To Go Home

# Wishing To Go Home

CATHERINE A. SHARP

Copyright © 2023 by Catherine A. Sharp.

Library of Congress Control Number: 2023919184
ISBN: Hardcover 979-8-3694-9364-9
Softcover 979-8-3694-9362-5
eBook 979-8-3694-9363-2

All rights reserved. No part of this book may be reproduced or transmitted in any form or by any means, electronic or mechanical, including photocopying, recording, or by any information storage and retrieval system, without permission in writing from the copyright owner.

Any people depicted in stock imagery provided by Getty Images are models, and such images are being used for illustrative purposes only.
Certain stock imagery © Getty Images.

Print information available on the last page.

Rev. date: 10/27/2023

**To order additional copies of this book, contact:**
Xlibris
844-714-8691
www.Xlibris.com
Orders@Xlibris.com
855059

The fifth Australian Aged Care Employee Day

7 August 2023

'Thanks for Caring'

# CONTENTS

Dedication..................................................................ix
Disclaimer .................................................................xi
Preface....................................................................xiii
Acknowledgements.................................................xv

Your Gut Feelings – Trust Them! ................................ 1
What Does It All Mean? ............................................... 7
What Can, Or Should, You Do To Help? ..................... 9
Power Of Attorney (POA) ...........................................11
Aged Care Assessment............................................... 13
Finding An Aged Care Facility – A 'Home' ................ 16
Person-Centred Care ................................................. 20
Sleep And Sleep Deprivation ..................................... 22
Becoming Involved In The Facility ............................ 24
What Is An Advanced Care Directive? ......................27
What To Tell Individual Staff Members ..................... 29
The End....................................................................... 31

About The Author ......................................................33
My First Visit To A Residential Aged Care Facility ..........37
Some Of My Qualifications Include:.......................... 41
Some Of My Publications Include: ............................ 41

# DEDICATION

This book is dedicated to my darling Mother. We had such a close, loving, chatty relationship over many wonderful years. We would talk for hours and hours at a time, over lunch, out shopping and on the phone in the evenings. Without sharing so much with her in her later years, I would never have learnt so much, felt so much, dealt with so much and this book would never have been written.

My parents lived in a lovely Benevolent Society retirement village in Sydney, for many years. They had lots of friends. They had barbeques, did the gardening together, went on holidays, outings to cafes, and to dancing. My Father did not dance but my Mother certainly did and it kept her so fit.

Later, some years after my Father had died, my Mother went to a locked dementia unit where she lived with 11 other ambulant women. I never saw any of them talking to each other. Even when they sat in the dining room together, they did not speak to each other. My Mother did not make friends with any of the other women. They all seemed to be lost in their own world of dementia.

When she could no longer walk I took her to a nursing home where she spent her last months. The nursing home was old, but it was warm and there was always music playing. The staff, who were all gorgeous, would put Mum, and the other residents, in recliner chairs in front of a giant television to watch old musicals from the 1930s and 1940s. My Mother was so happy listening to them. I could see that. She always had a smile, even though she could no longer communicate with me. I think she always knew who I was though.

# DISCLAIMER

The information in this book is very general and taken from personal experience as well as my own experience as a registered nurse working in hospitals, the community and residential aged care facilities. It is not set in stone, merely to give people some information about ageing, forgetfulness, loss of mobility, dementia, and ideas to consider. I offer suggestions based on my own experiences with ageing parents, and residents, about rights, possibilities, and options. I offer suggestions based on my decades of nursing which included visiting 200 or so residential aged care facilities in Sydney as a Wound Care Consultant over many years. The services described may not be available or applicable in all countries.

# PREFACE

I have written this book for when I grow old; for when I need help, can no longer drive, cut my toenails, manage my money, shop, cook, clean, or remember to eat and shower. It is for when, heaven forbid, I can no longer communicate with anyone, verbally. If I cannot make you understand me, and I cannot understand you, how will we know what to do. How will I shop, do the banking, pay bills?

It is for my children and grandchildren, so they'll know what to do when the time comes; so that they'll know what I want, where to find things, jobs to do, finances to take over. In past generations discussions about finance and planning for death just did not occur. Those days are gone, and I think all family members would be much better off if they discussed the subject of dying and death as easily as if they were planning a picnic in a park.

It is for all my friends whose parents are ageing and who want to know what to do for the best; knowing there is no time to waste. What if they have a stroke tomorrow and cannot speak, or write, or remember. It is for every great-grandparent, grandparent, parent, child, niece, nephew, grand-child, great grand-child, aunts and uncles and cousins, for every single family. And it is for every nurse caring for the aged, whether you are the boss, the Registered Nurse, the Assistant in Nursing or Personal

Care Assistant, the Doctor, the bus driver, the person serving you in the local corner shop, the kitchen hand or cleaning lady....no matter what job you do.

It is for Faculties of Nursing, Social Sciences, Medicine, and Law in any University anywhere in the world. It is for Colleges teaching care staff. It is about providing consent for treatment you may not know anything about until your loved one is in care. It is to provide you all with some understanding of what it might be like to be elderly, to have a stroke, to suffer from memory loss and dementia and what it is like to be unable to communicate normally with you.

I want to give you some insight into some behavioural changes that may occur because of memory loss or dementia and to offer some tips for you to help you deal with the process, the illness.

Each time I visited my Mother, firstly in her Benevolent Society retirement village, then in the dementia facility, then the nursing home which was virtually every day, at different times of the day, I learnt something new about her ageing process and her view of the future as she prepared herself for the end...not that she always wanted to die but sometimes she would tell me she thought the time was getting closer.

I have a much clearer vision of what she 'saw' in her future on the other side...and it is not to be feared at all.

# ACKNOWLEDGEMENTS

I do want to thank the Benevolent Society in Sydney for all the friends my parents made when living in their retirement village, all the activities, the exercise equipment and library, the bus trips, and the help and kindness that Mum and I received when my Father died. Then later when I needed support and advice when Mum had her stroke and slowly developed dementia... Thank you.

I also dedicate this book to the wonderful care staff who looked after my Mother in both the dementia facility, then the nursing home where she was transferred to when she became bedridden and where she died.

The photograph on the front cover is my Mother walking into the residential aged care facility dementia unit with my eldest son, after a long walk. Thank you to my four wonderful children for helping with both my parents but especially with Mum after Dad's death.

"Oh, when are you coming to get me?" whispered my Mother as she looked up at the sky; pale blue with cotton-ball clouds. 'What do you mean?' I asked (but my breaking heart already knew). She couldn't see the tears welling up behind my sunglasses, but she couldn't see very well anyway. She had macular degeneration.

"I want to know when they are coming to get me...you know...when am I going to die?"

That day we were doing what we did every week at the end of my visit to her retirement village. After my Father died Mum continued living there until she went into care. She would always walk me out to my car and stand and wave till I drove off and was out of sight. We hugged even longer that day. Every week I would visit Mum and take fresh salmon, a favourite of hers. I would make a salad and we'd spend the day chatting. It became a ritual when she no longer wanted to go out.

She'd talk about her youth, dancing, sleeping on Blackpool beach as a naughty teenager, and the love of her life, my Father, a Scottish soldier.

She told me about the dreams she had, regularly, about having dinner with her deceased parents and three brothers, one of whom had died when he was five from a 'blockage' in his stomach. She described how his coffin was left open in the living room of their home in England and the smell of soap ...people would walk through to pay their respects to this dear little boy.

The dreams about having dinner with her parents and her brothers, who were all dead, told me that she believed in a life beyond this one, and she was genuinely looking forward to seeing them all again.

I drove off but stopped around the corner. I just had to park the car and I howled...and sobbed noisily...and howled. This happened every time I left her. As hard as that was it opened up a whole new topic, dying and death, hard to think about but it became easy, and completely normal, each time we were together. I knew exactly what she wanted when the time came.

# YOUR GUT FEELINGS
# – TRUST THEM!

If you are lucky enough to see your ageing relative on a regular basis you will know that all is not good if:

They were always smartly dressed and would never dream of wearing the same outfit several days in a row, but now they have the same outfit on day after day.

The clothes look a bit grubby...you know...egg yolk on their tie, tea drips on a shirt.

They have bad breath...perhaps teeth are not being cleaned...dentures not being removed.

Not walking as much because 'feet are sore'.

The fresh salad you made a week ago is grey and furry on the table.

There's a bar of soap in the fridge and pantyhose in the bread bin.

The milk (now very 'off') is in the cupboard not the fridge.

All the plates (usually kept in the cupboard) are missing -- look in the oven.

There is no garbage to take out; no empty packets, no vegetable scraps, no empty milk cartons…a sign they may not be eating at all.

They have always showered, got dressed and made their bed first thing in the morning, washed the dishes after every meal, but one day you visit and they are still in their nightclothes, dishes piled in the sink and the bed is unmade.

You see the glass chopping board on the bathroom floor! This is terrifying especially when they cannot see it or tell you why they have put it there.

You know something is wrong, even if you don't really know what.

But then the worst thing happened…my Mother phoned me one morning and when I answered I said, "Oh Mum it sounds like you have a really bad cold". I called an ambulance and drove to her home. I was sure she was having a stroke just by the tone in her voice. I arrived as the paramedics were walking her from her house to the ambulance. I was thinking, and hoping, that if it was a stroke, it must be mild…because she was 88 years old and walking quite normally! How wrong I was.

Mum was hospitalised for five weeks and treated appallingly by some nursing staff. I did not see this of course but found out from other women in her four-bed room when I visited. The ward was very short-staffed and because I am a hospital-trained registered nurse I could see the problem. The nurses were unable to care for my Mother safely. One night she fell out of bed, landing on her head, and I only found out when I asked why she had a big bruise on her forehead. It was not the staff who told me but the other patients, the ladies in her room.

She recovered quite well, then when I brought her home after this five-week hospital stay she walked in her front door and let out an incredulous gasp. 'What have you done with all my things?' she yelped. I had, of course, done nothing with her things.

Everything was the same as five weeks before when she was hospitalised. 'Where is my bath? What have you done with my bath?' 'You took my bath out and put a shower there instead!'

But this was just the beginning. This was vascular dementia...the very sad, dreadful confusion...the suspicion, the paranoia, and the accusations. She could not be left alone again all the time, so we arranged for a beautiful carer to visit each day to help her with food, medications, and to take her for a long walk. She loved walking, but I could see she would never be able to care for herself in her retirement village anymore even though she was physically quite fit. She had been a dancer all her life. She had forgotten how to use her microwave, she put paper in her oven, forgot to put her milk back in the fridge, forgot to take her pills, left her front door wide open. She was once found by a neighbour outside her home in the dark of night, just standing and staring at the moon. I felt this might be the beginnings of wandering, a terrifying thought. Old people with dementia can go missing completely!

Mum had a lovely doctor who she had been seeing for many years and she did confirm the vascular dementia following her stroke. I knew it, but was in such denial mainly because she was still dancing with friends every day.

Talking to Mum about going into care was easy some days and I would book a visit to take her to see facilities but when I arrived to pick her up, she refused to go so I'd have to cancel that visit. Anyway, one day she did agree to go to a facility near where I lived, just for a few days...or that was the plan.

I booked her into respite care for a brief period in a 12-bed locked dementia unit. She never left, never went home again. She was so unhappy, her dementia got worse, but she lived there for many months. The care staff were lovely, but I could see there was never enough staff. On the afternoon / evening shift there was only ever one care worker. I was there with Mum most days, at different times and I would help her to undress for bed and encourage her to clean her teeth. I often had to do them for her and that was a 20-minute ritual. It is not possible for one care worker to clean the teeth of 12 residents when it takes 20-minutes for each---that is four hours, just spent cleaning teeth.

Anyone with responsibility for caring for our aged and frail-aged is dreaming if they think the care staff can give optimum care to even 12 residents. Often, they are charged with caring for many, many more. They are responsible for showering, changing incontinence pads, ensuring food is served and eaten, giving out medications etc. etc. so accidents happen. Residents fall over. They may be unable to get up. We cannot expect one care worker to lift a resident off the ground alone. What if the resident fractures a femur? Who will help?

I received a telephone call early one morning from the night duty carer, in the facility, telling me my Mother had fallen during the night. Imagine my shock when I asked who was looking after her in the locked dementia unit overnight and was told 'nobody'. There was one female care worker for 46 residents in this two-storey facility and she remained upstairs all night. So, my Mother and 11 other women, all with dementia, were locked in to one part of the facility with nobody looking after them.

Over a period of years visiting residential aged care facilities, as a Wound Care Nurse Consultant, I found out that it was not unusual to leave the aged and demented locked up and alone all night. But it was the one question I did not ask management when I put my Mother into care. I never thought to ask how many staff are on night duty? What was the staff resident ratio? How could management of this facility be at ease with themselves, knowing there was only one care worker to look after 46 residents, some in wheelchairs and physically dependant on just one staff member to help. There should have been two staff at the very least, to help lift and transfer the less mobile residents to the toilet for example. And what if a fight started between residents in the locked dementia unit? Residents could kill each other and if the carer went to intervene, he or she could have been bashed unconscious. This has happened in other facilities. If there is only one carer it means they do not get any official break times. The carers are unlikely to speak out because they may no longer have a job if they do!

Carers told me a lot of things they were concerned about, but they did not want me to mention their names to the Director of Nursing at this facility. I was concerned that the alarm did not go off to alert the carer upstairs that my Mother had fallen. She was 'found' on the floor. I was told when Mum entered this dementia unit that there were movement sensors that would alert staff, but care staff told me something different. The sensors were not working and had not worked for ages. Care staff had told management.

# WHAT DOES IT ALL MEAN?

The person who was always smartly dressed may be wearing the same outfit two or more days in a row because they are no longer able to wash and hang out clothes. Perhaps they are sleeping in their clothes...forgetting to get undressed at the end of the day.

If there is egg yolk on their tie, or tea drips on their blouse it may be because they cannot see very well.

Bad breath could mean they are forgetting to clean their teeth and / or they may have tooth decay. Having tooth decay means there is a chance they will not eat, or not eat enough, because it is too painful.

Sore feet could mean they have long, curly toenails and can no longer see them or cut them. Sometimes they put their shoes on the wrong feet.

Food that they have put in the fridge is a huge worry when you see that it is wild, grey, and furry. If they have poor vision, they may not see it and eat it.

Finding a bar of soap in the fridge, or pantyhose in the bread bin means they are suffering from confused thoughts.

Finding an open carton of milk in the cupboard instead of the fridge is a huge worry because they may drink 'off' milk and become violently ill.

If the plates are not in the usual place try looking in the oven, or bedroom wardrobe.

If there is no garbage it could mean they are not eating, yet if you ask them, they will tell you they have 'just eaten'.

# WHAT CAN, OR SHOULD, YOU DO TO HELP?

Ask the person's doctor for a referral to a psycho-geriatrician; somebody who specialises in dementia.

You do not want to take away their independence, yet you know their day-to-day life may be getting quite dangerous. You can see, or sense, the risks, and sometimes their friends will tell you they are worried about them.

It may be that soon they will either need to go into a care facility or will need full-time care in their own home. Can they live with you? Do they even want to live with you.

You just want them to be safe.

Offer to wash their clothes for them.

Arrange for a housekeeper / carer who could clean, wash, vacuum, dust and shop for food.

Book an appointment with their dentist and take them. If decay is found, or an abscess or loose teeth it can be very painful, and the pain will prevent them from chewing their food. This could lead to insufficient nutrition.

Phone a podiatrist and set up regular home visits or take them to a podiatrist. This will ensure their feet are kept in perfect order. This is vital for anyone whose eyesight is fading. They cannot cut their own toenails safely. This is important for diabetics who may have peripheral neuropathy, which means loss of feeling, loss of sensation in the feet. A cut can become infected resulting in amputation.

Offer to clean out the fridge for them and / or just do it while you are making coffee. You can check whether the milk is fresh enough to drink (look at the date as well) and look for wild, grey, furry, foods or anything that looks off and just 'bin it'.

Every time I visited Mum when she was still living at home, over the years after my Father died, I would take the garbage out to the bin as I left. The garbage bag was always full, good evidence that she was eating. There were empty 'meals on wheels' packets, biscuit wrappers, tea bags, and milk cartons. Then one day there was much less in her garbage.

The days old meal is still in the fridge when you visit. The bottle of orange juice bought a fortnight before had 'blown' and was about to explode.

A neighbour returns their wheelie-walker that was left in the car park or round at the local corner shop...again!

# POWER OF ATTORNEY (POA)

It can be very difficult for any family member, a son or daughter, a spouse or adult grandchild, to find that not only is their beloved relative's memory fading but they are forgetting important things, and nobody has POA to help, or take over.

Firstly, I must advise you to talk to a lawyer long before their memory starts to fade. You may be advised to draw up a will. I am not qualified to advise here but I was so fortunate that my Father had a will before he died and he made me executrix. He was always a very organised man, and I did not have to do anything when he died.

Likewise, I did not have to do anything when my Mother died. She had a will and a lawyer who dealt with everything. My Mother asked me if I would take on the role of POA some years before her death when she was still independent and very fit, dancing every day and walking miles.

We went to her solicitor together and I signed the POA forms then we went to her bank so I could meet her bank manager and the POA forms were photocopied and put on file. I had no idea what holding POA meant but became very knowledgeable and learned to manage her financial affairs for her...thank goodness.

For me it was an enormous learning experience because my parents never talked about money. That was, for that generation, a subject never discussed. It was taboo. Learning about Mum's finances was something that evolved over time as she became more and more visually impaired, and she would ask me to read her mail for her. Only then did I start to find out what she had and what I then had to deal with.

But in the couple of years before she went into a dementia unit, I realised she did not know who she banked with, or how many bank accounts she had, and in which countries!

Keep an eye open for overdue bills, mail from overseas, and insurance that needs renewal. You may find that important mail has been put in a 'safe place' and this requires you to deal with it...phone calls, explanations, cancellations. What I did, and this was just one good solution for me, was to have all Mum's mail redirected to me, so that nothing got overlooked. I paid her bills on time and discontinued subscriptions to magazines. She could no longer see to be able to read them anyway.

I suggest that it is a good idea to let your children know all of this, as much as you want to share with them before you lose your memory. Don't leave your possessions, money, estate, to be 'discovered' after you are gone. I gave all my children and my best friend, a copy of my will, years ago. My children have met my lawyer. I want to make it easy for everybody.

# AGED CARE ASSESSMENT

When you just 'know' that your ageing parent is not coping so well, forgetting to put the milk in the fridge, forgetting to eat, forgetting to pay bills, or change clothes, it may be time to chat with their doctor. These are all routine daily tasks that they have performed for decades, and you are now worried about their safety, so it is a great idea to have a chat with somebody from an Aged Care Assessment Team (ACAT). They will no doubt have a different name in every country, but their purpose will be the same.

The ACAT are multi-disciplinary, and their role is to inform and advise families and carers, as well as the elderly themselves, to make informed decisions about care they'll require in the future.

Talk to your relative's doctor. Each country may have different referral methods. An ACAT assessment and approval may be a mandatory requirement before you can request government subsidised residential aged care, community care or extended aged care at home packages. Again, every State, Territory and country will be different.

Some of the options I discussed with the ACAT were firstly, getting a carer to come to Mum's home because she did not want to leave home and go into a residential aged care facility. This proved to be an excellent arrangement for a while. The carer would take Mum for an hour-long walk, do her shopping with her, or for her, prepare her lunch and ensure she took her pills. The carer would phone me with concerns and leave comments/requests in an exercise book at Mum's home.

One thing that worried me about her showering alone was that even though she wore a 'falls alarm' around her neck Mum always took it off and hung it on the back of the bathroom door. I never convinced her to keep it on in the shower. I kept telling her that it was waterproof and designed to be always worn – even in the shower!

The ACAT assisted by working out the most appropriate level of care that would best meet Mum's needs when the time was right. They helped me to find a suitable home for her. In Australia the ACAT can provide interpreters if required. Again, each country may have other options.

The ACAT were there for me when I felt a bit fragile, having to deal with Mum's needs. I have total confidence in recommending their services. They took a huge weight off my shoulders.

My Mother went dancing with all her friends several days a week before she had a stroke. It was a mild stroke, but it certainly affected her over a period of three years or so, albeit slowly. Her physical state was fine, and she continued to dance and walk for miles every day. She spent almost every day with friends in her retirement village and with her grandchildren and great grandchildren at the weekend and in school holidays.

She was philosophical about dying as was my Father and long before they died they went with friends from the retirement village to the local cemetery to choose 'holes in the wall' so they could be together after death. I thought that was a lovely idea!

# FINDING AN AGED CARE FACILITY – A 'HOME'

## What to look for and questions to ask

If you are unfamiliar with residential aged care facilities, you may wish to talk to your ACAT. I chose to bring my Mother to a facility close to where I lived. This also meant that she would be close to her grandchildren and great grandchildren.

Mum had always said that even though she wanted to stay at home, if she really had to go into care, she wanted her own room and an ensuite bathroom. So, I started looking around and some of the facilities I looked at I had been to on several occasions in my role as a Wound Care Consultant to see residents with wounds.

The facility I chose for Mum was small and I had been there on a few occasions. The staff seemed really nice, and, on the day I phoned, the Director told me that he had a single room available so I booked it quick-smart before somebody else did.

There are several things to look for and ask about and they are not really in any specific order. You must keep in mind the mobility of the relative / resident going into care. My Mother was incredibly lucky to be so agile and mobile after a lifetime of dancing. She was little, five feet and two inches, and weighed less than 50 kgs and she was very flexible. When my children were young, they used to say she was the only Granny who could run all the way around a soccer field. She walked every single day, often for many miles, and she danced and danced and danced.

**Things You May Consider:**

Are there stairs inside and outside the building?

Is there a lift? Is it big enough to get an ambulance trolley in to transport a resident in the event they do fall and fracture a femur.

Is access good and easy?

Is there wheelchair access?

Is there a medical centre and hospital close by?

Are the toilet seats raised?

Advice from the retirement villages / nursing homes associations (they may be called something different in your country).

Is there lovely music playing? Is the music appropriate for the age of the residents? Is the music in the language suitable for the residents?

Are the staff multilingual? They do not all have to speak English.

What is the atmosphere like…by that I mean I wanted to feel the warmth, the calm, see a caring manager. I wanted to see how the manager talked to the residents and the staff. Was s/he polite and respectful to the staff. How did the nurses and care staff speak to the residents and each other? Were they all calm and peaceful?

How was the ambient temperature? Was the heating on? Or was there a howling gale whistling through the building?

Does the manager understand that your elderly relative may be terrified? Terrified of leaving his or her home to come into a dementia unit? Did s/he understand what I wanted and how sad and protective I was feeling?

You probably won't be told that residents may wake up when other residents are screaming, or entering their rooms, frightening the living daylights out of them. You probably won't be told that your loved relative may or may not go back to sleep after being woken. You will not be told that whether wide awake or not they may be showered at five in the morning ready for breakfast because that is what the care staff has been told to do.

You are not told that they will be so sleep-deprived for the rest of their days that they can never enjoy activities or outings. Even though they have a normal capability to sleep the regime will transform the pattern of their lives.

I went to see the facility and the vacant room was number 7, Mum's lucky number. There was lavender growing in the courtyard, a favourite flower.

Do they have a 'person-centred care' philosophy? What is that?

# PERSON-CENTRED CARE

My Mother was always a good sleeper before she entered care. She always told me, when she was still in the Benevolent Society village, that she'd sleep till eight in the morning then have two cups of very hot English tea. She would then have breakfast with more tea, then she'd shower and get ready for the day.

This seemed to work fine when she first went into care, and I believe the Director of the facility saw to it that she was left to sleep and wake up of her own accord. I don't know because to begin with I did not go in to visit her early in the morning. I did not want her woken at six in the morning. I wanted an assurance from management that Mum would not be woken and that she would be able to sleep until she woke naturally. If I asked her if she'd had a good sleep, she often could not tell me. She had forgotten and I began to realise that she was forgetting more and more things.

To begin with she was showered by staff in the mornings and nurses told me that she would scream the building down when the water started pouring all over her. I was distraught. She never had a problem showering at home and I did not want her to start her days screaming and feeling frightened, so I told the Director and staff not to shower her at all anymore.

Instead, I took in HiCare™ bath cloths, a disposable, complete, prepackaged bathing product. It is an Australian made product that replaces the traditional shower, or bed-bath.[1] I also provided beautiful, natural moisturising creams and a manicure set with lovely nail varnish. She loved having her nails done as did many of the residents in the facility.

I have seen, in some facilities, that staff would share nail varnish between several residents but that potentially puts all residents at risk of cross-infection. Sometimes, although it's an awful thought, residents have faeces under their fingernails. So, the way to prevent cross-infection is for each resident to have their own manicure kit with nail file, nail varnish and varnish remover.

---

[1] I am not, and never have been, paid by any company to promote their products.

# SLEEP AND SLEEP DEPRIVATION

You think your ageing relative is getting a good night's sleep and waking naturally, when they are ready to wake up, not being woken by staff and showered at five am. The lack of informed consent to waken residents to suit the staff's workload and the resultant unnecessary sleep deprivation, may contribute to behavioural problems. Regardless of dementia, the use of two-hourly repositioning to prevent pressure ulcers, is harmful, and residents with dementia have no ability to provide informed consent.

There are key gaps in the care of residents. Identifying a link between sleep deprivation and Alzheimer's disease and the medico-legal implications is fascinating and we nurses need to work with sleep scientists to ensure the scientific evidence for sleep will transcend to residents so that the traditional routine, entrenched in nursing care, is modified to suit individual residents. But what is clear is that this traditional nursing practice, of repositioning two-hourly, does wake many residents, causing sleep deprivation. I have read many reports about residents who 'became aggressive when woken at night to be repositioned'.

I have never seen any evidence in the literature to recommend a regimen of two-hourly repositioning because pressure ulcers can occur with just an hour of unrelieved pressure on any tissue that lies between the bony skeleton and the mattress or chair cushion.

Sleep deprivation may contribute to challenging behaviours and is an unnecessary breach of human rights that occurs without informed consent. I have seen many residents who were, I believe, severely sleep deprived. It is evident when residents are asleep at the breakfast table because they are continually woken by noise or woken to be showered, yet they just want to lie down and sleep. Waking residents may be considered 'unintentional institutional' abuse. I have known of residential aged care facilities that wake residents from sleep every two hours to go to the toilet! This is outrageous. The pads for incontinent residents have, for many years, been able to absorb a gallon of urine and the beds do not get wet. Let them sleep...please! When these residents are wearing incontinence pads nothing disastrous will happen. We can improve the care for our aged and frail aged with or without a diagnosis of dementia with much better outcomes.

# BECOMING INVOLVED IN THE FACILITY

One way to make sure Mum was eating well was to go in at mealtimes to help. I used to go in the evenings after work and seeing how busy the one care worker was would just horrify me. S/he would have to dish out soup that was so hot it was dangerous. The temperature of the soup was supposed to be recorded by staff, but I never saw a thermometer being used. I offered to take the temperature of the soup but was told there was no thermometer. Why did it have to be scalding hot? It became a habit going in to help with the evening meal, serve and clean up, while chatting to my Mother and the other residents. It was a locked dementia unit and many of the residents were non-verbal. If you don't understand the workload, it is very rewarding to volunteer. You may have to sign up to become an official volunteer so ask the Director of Care what you must do.

One of the saddest things for me was to find that I was frequently the only visiting relative in the dementia unit. What would you do if somebody was scalded with soup? What are staff supposed to do? One of the strangest things, I feel, is that none of the residents in the dementia unit had any identifying features, no wrist labels, no visible labels on clothing, so if an agency nurse is on duty, they have no way of knowing the names of the residents. Few of these residents could tell you their own name. Most could not communicate at all. When it came time for the nurse to give out the medications, which they dispensed from a Webster pack, it really was a guessing game as to which medications belonged to which resident...very scary. Nobody would know who had had what medications because many residents did not know their own names. If you said 'Hello Edith' they may all answer, or perhaps nobody will answer.

One thing to look for when you are visiting is the way medications are given. Having all pills in Webster packs individually labelled is the safest way to dispense...if you know the names of the residents.

But one evening I was visiting Mum and I took her to the dining room and joined her at the table. I did not eat because the facility was not set up to provide food for visitors and that was fine. I was the only visitor there that evening and I used to go regularly to make sure Mum had a good appetite and was eating well.

On this evening, to my horror, I watched a care worker walking around the dining room with a tray full of little pots into which she had 'popped' everybody's pills; pills for all 12 women that is. The Webster packs were nowhere to be seen! When the nurse got to Mum's dining table, she gave some pills out then walked to the next table.

"Do you have Mum's pills?" I asked the care worker. She froze with a look of terror. She knew I was a registered nurse, as did all the staff. What you have just done, I told her, the way you have given the pills out is absolutely against all the rules and you know, or should, know that. How do you know what pills you have given to what resident? You know I will have to report you to the Director.

"I didn't pop them out of the Webster pack she said... somebody else did that before I took over".

The risk of making a mistake and giving the wrong medication to the wrong resident, because of this practice, was huge. I reported this care worker to the Director the next morning and she was taken out of the dementia unit straight away.

But imagine my horror when the same thing happened a few days later with another nurse! This was clearly a common, accepted practice in this facility and for staff to break the rules like this with medication was horrifying.

And what if a resident collapsed, or fell and broke a bone? Well, I hope they all have an Advanced Care Directive (ACD).

# WHAT IS AN ADVANCED CARE DIRECTIVE?

This is a form authorising somebody else to make decisions for you if you are too sick or unable to decide for yourself. I think it is vital to have discussions firstly with the person who will / may be going into care or who is already in a nursing home for example. Do not wait until they have a diagnosis of dementia.

If you can talk about it when you and other family members are all together having lunch for example, then you'll make the right decision if the elderly family member loses capacity. My Mother found this very easy to talk about and she was ready to go...she had no fear of dying. She gave me clear instructions.

Find out what they want if for example they get a shocking cold. Do they just want to be given warm lemon juice and a box of tissues or do they want the doctor to be called? If they have a fall and fracture a femur, then the facility must call an ambulance. But if they collapse, unconscious, and have no palpable pulse then staff must know whether to start CPR and call an ambulance or just wait with them as they die. That may be just a matter of minutes.

There are many scenarios you can probably think of. It may be that nurses call the family who may wish to gather around the bed and wait for that last breath. If there is no

ACD somebody may, with all good intent, start CPR and call an ambulance. Doing CPR can result in fractured ribs and if the resident is transferred to hospital, they may have tubes inserted into every orifice and life may be prolonged when it really shouldn't be.

A copy of the ACD should be kept with the primary doctor, family members, the Aged Care Facility and every member of staff in that facility should know who wants what, as far as the ACD goes.

# WHAT TO TELL INDIVIDUAL STAFF MEMBERS

Care staff are constantly busy, and their heads are full of things they must do for residents from cleaning teeth to checking hearing aids are in and working, to showering, changing pads, cleaning up incontinent residents and cutting up food for those who cannot do it themselves. So, there is no way we can expect them to remember detailed instructions about our relatives and every resident they are caring for on the day. They will not know what every resident wants in the event of a nasty cold, a fall, a head injury, a fractured femur, or a complete collapse, with loss of consciousness and /or death. Do they want CPR? What are care staff supposed to do? There is no time to go to the office and look up the notes for an ACD.

You may see relatives on each side of the bed, one screaming 'Do everything you can!!!! Another saying… 'No CPR… she does not want that.'

Here is a suggestion. It is what I did with, and for, staff in Mum's facility. Often, I took packets of biscuits, lollies and chocolate for all the staff and in her last weeks of life I would chat with the staff and just say… 'You know Mum is not for resuscitation.' Often, they would not know those details because they are just too busy. The subject may not be broached in clinical handovers and even if it was staff cannot be expected to remember every detail of care for 50 or more residents. And there's a staff turnover to consider too. That is different in every facility.

On the morning that she died Mum had been showered and dressed and was having breakfast when she just died in her chair. Staff put her back into bed and called me. I raced into the nursing home and although I was devastated beyond belief, I was so happy to see her in bed, fully dressed. Staff had put a rose on her pillow. There was no CPR, just as I had wanted. There was no ambulance. It was all that she wanted --- a very peaceful passing.

# THE END

When Mum was admitted to the locked dementia unit, I told the nurses I would be taking her washing home. I would do that for my Mother because in the days we spent together, when she was still living at home and could think and act for herself, she used to tell me that if she ever had to go in to residential aged care I was to wash her clothes for her. She did not want her clothes to go into a washing machine with other people's clothes.

So, we had a sign typed on an A4 sheet, laminated, and stuck onto Mum's wardrobe.

It read: **'ALL WASHING TO GO HOME'**.
One day soon after moving in, my Mother
was quite upset, and as she was
pacing around her room she saw the sign.
She walked closer to the wardrobe
and peered at the words for just a
moment...then shouted at me:

'Yes, I *am* wishing to go home'.

And now she is home.

My Mother died in July 2012 aged 91.

# ABOUT THE AUTHOR

I was born in Airthrey Castle in Stirling, Scotland. My father was a Scottish soldier stationed at Stirling Castle and my parents lived in the married quarters in King Stables Lane. We moved to Kenya when I was five, during the Mau-Mau Uprising (1952–1960), also known as the Mau Mau Rebellion, the Kenya Emergency, and the Mau Mau Revolt, a war in the British Kenya Colony. It was here that I was taken to visit an African hospital by a friend of my parents who was a nurse working at the hospital. Overcrowding was rampant, and patients were waiting to be seen, sitting on the dry dusty earth outside in the burning hot sun. That sight is imprinted in my memory.

I always wanted to be a nurse and I think the visit to that hospital in Kenya influenced me greatly.

I lived in Germany for five years and attended Queens School, Rheindahlen. I left school when I was 16 years of age to start work as a nurse's aide, on the children's ward, at the Royal Air Force Hospital in Wegberg, Germany. I then moved to England with my family and began my hospital-based training as a nurse, in Sheffield, Yorkshire, in 1965. I studied a combined children's and general nursing course for four years beginning with 18 months of training at Western Bank Children's Hospital. This wonderful hospital was a specialist centre for newborns upwards with spina bifida and hydrocephalus, all at risk of pressure ulcers because they could not reposition themselves or feel the pain of pressure. I do not remember seeing pressure ulcers in these little ones.

I then switched to general training for 18 months in the Sheffield Royal Infirmary, an old hospital with long open 'Nightingale Wards' and beds down each side of the wards. It was physically demanding work. The junior nurses worked in pairs all day and through the night repositioning ('turning') patients every two hours to prevent pressure ulcers. Night duty staff had most patients sitting up for breakfast and day staff would start 'turning' patients at eight o'clock in the morning. We would begin with the patients in bed number one, work down one side of the ward and up the other, flipping patients over onto their right or left side. This took about two hours. We signed the charts at the foot of the bed, as there were no computers at that time, to indicate the time we had turned patients, and which side they were lying on, right or left, then repeated the process. We 'flipped' everyone over every two hours, so that by mealtimes everyone was sitting upright. This ritual happened throughout the 24 hours.

Interestingly I do not remember the term 'dementia' in the 1960's nor do I remember nursing, or seeing, old patients. I think 60 would have been the oldest. I had never heard of residential aged care facilities.

I returned to Western Bank Children's Hospital to finish the fourth year of training, then became a children's staff nurse at Thornbury Annexe for a year before emigrating to Australia.

I began working in the Intensive Care Unit at the Royal Hobart Hospital, Tasmania, and do not remember seeing any patients with pressure ulcers, nor do I remember the term 'dementia'.

The practice of two-hourly repositioning was, unsurprisingly, the mainstay of pressure ulcer prevention. This ritual started with Florence Nightingale on her wards, which revealed structural similarities with the Sheffield Royal Infirmary. It also took Florence two hours to go down one side of the ward and up the other 'turning' patients. It is said that she blamed nurses if patients developed pressure ulcers. This mode of blame continues to this day, with nurses and care staff frequently blamed for pressure ulcer development, by staff who do not understand that pressure ulcers can develop in less than 30 minutes in immobile patients, yet they are powerless to prevent them.

About 1997 I created my own business, The Wound Centre, so that I could see residents privately in their homes or in residential aged care facilities. As well as seeing patients with surgical site infections in Royal Prince Alfred Hospital, I was frequently asked to see patients who had pressure ulcers because of immobility, either during surgery or following a stroke or fractured femur.

It was clear to me that not only was two-hourly repositioning not sufficient or successful, but that nobody, nurses, or doctors, could see what I saw. They did not understand me, when I said these patients need to be on an alternating pressure air mattress which would, more likely than not, prevent pressure ulcers. So, I was baffled as to why they were not being used at this or any other major Sydney hospital.

I was seeing patients with pressure ulcers. I was reporting these pressure ulcers. Denial from management was difficult to understand and it was with some exasperation on their part that I was charged with the job of investigating these pressure ulcers further. Regardless, my wound care role was about to expand beyond this hospital to residential aged care facilities.

# MY FIRST VISIT TO A RESIDENTIAL AGED CARE FACILITY

In 1997, while working full-time at the Royal Prince Alfred Hospital, Sydney I received a call from a general practitioner who asked if I could see a resident with a sacral pressure ulcer in a residential aged care facility. I had never been to a residential aged care facility and certainly did not know if Royal Prince Alfred Hospital management would let me go, so I did not ask, nor did I ever tell them. I went after hours, met the resident, and her daughter, also a nurse, and the care staff who were so kind to the resident and so helpful to me.

I began to receive more and more requests from the doctors and Directors of Nursing in residential aged care facilities to see residents with wounds, and to teach staff. I loved it. I went after hours and sometimes at weekends. From that day in 1997 till 2020 I visited around 200 residential aged care facilities all over Sydney, from Kuringai to Manly, to Bankstown and the Sutherland Shire. I went to some facilities just once but many I visited on a regular basis to see the same residents, see the progress, or lack of, with their wounds, meet the families, and discuss potential investigations and treatment with the doctors.

During these years I was also contracted to work with a Community Nursing Service in Northern Sydney. There were six centres, and I would arrange to meet nurses outside the homes of clients with wounds. Then I'd go in with the nurses who would introduce me to the clients and give me a history of their wounds, whether a post-operative wound dehiscence or an ulcer on the sole of the foot from diabetic peripheral neuropathy.

The nurse would open the dressing pack, sometimes on the floor, depending on where the client was sitting or lying. Often, we'd have to 'shoo away' the cat so that it did not walk all over the forceps and cotton balls! Some homes were immaculately clean but others not so much. On more than one occasion I had permission from management to order an alternating pressure air mattress for a bedridden client at home.

Many managers of aged care facilities were open to my suggestion of nursing bedridden residents on an alternating pressure air mattress[2] to prevent pressure ulcers from developing even though residents' pressure ulcers never healed as far as I could see. Residents still died with pressure ulcers. It was disturbing to find out that staff were still repositioning residents two-hourly even when residents were on an alternating pressure air mattress. This was a force of habit but should never have been done as it defeated the purpose of having an alternating pressure air mattress. I was very concerned about residents being woken when they were repositioned.

---

[2] The Nodec A alternating pressure air mattress was a favourite of mine. I am not, and never have been, paid by any company to promote products.

Since 1997, I have visited 200, or perhaps more, residential aged care facilities, seen hundreds of residents with wounds, and dementia. I have met the most enthusiastic nurses and care staff. I last saw a resident with a shocking wound in a residential aged care facility, in January 2020. I may never go into another residential aged care facility because of the rules around Covid that prohibit me from entering any residential aged care facility.

## SOME OF MY QUALIFICATIONS INCLUDE:

A PhD (Flinders Uni SA), Master of Health Law (USyd), a Master of Research in Public Health (UNSW), a Master of Clinical Nursing (USyd), State Registered Nurse and Registered Sick Children's Nurse (UK).

The only good thing about being locked down for the last three years was the amount of (extra) writing I was able to do. The last three publications on the list below were written in 2022. But altogether they do show that I have had an interest in dementia, the aged, pressure ulcers, skin tears, and sleep deprivation for more than 20 years.

## SOME OF MY PUBLICATIONS INCLUDE:

My PhD thesis is entitled 'Preventing Pressure Ulcers: Researching the Consequences of two-hourly repositioning without consent'. Flinders University, Humanities, Arts and Social Sciences, South Australia

Sharp CA, Burr G, Broadbent M, Cummins M, Casey H & Merriman A. Pressure Ulcer Prevention and Care: a survey of current practice. Journal of Quality in Clinical Practice. 2000 20: 150-157 htpps://doi.10.1046/j.1440-1762.2000.00384.x

Sharp CA and McLaws M-L. A discourse on pressure ulcer physiology: the implications of repositioning and staging. 2005 World Wide Wounds. http://www.worldwidewounds.com/2005/october/Sharp/Discourse-OnPressure-Ulcer-Physiology.html

Sharp CA, Burr G, Broadbent M, Cummins M, Casey H and Merriman A. Clinical variance in assessing risk of pressure ulcer development. British Journal of Nursing 2005 14(6) pp. S4-S12 https://www.proquest.com/docview/199474317

Sharp CA and McLaws M-L. Estimating the risk of pressure ulcer development: is it truly evidence-based? International Wound Journal December 2006 Volume 3 Issue 4 Page 344 – 353 https://doi:10.1111/j.1742- 481X.2006.00261.x

Sharp CA, White R, Ousey KJ, Butcher M & Iverson C. 'Response to Moore Z & Cowman S (2012) Pressure ulcer prevalence and prevention practices in care of the older person in the Republic of Ireland, Journal of Clinical Nursing 21, 362-371. J Clin Nurs 2012 Apr;21(7-8)vv:1191-2. https://10.1111/j.1365-2702.2011.04045.x

Sharp CA and White R. Pressure Ulcer Risk Assessment: Do we need a golden hour? Journal of Wound Care vol 24, no 3, March 2015 https://10.12968/jowc.2015.24.5.237

Sharp CA, Schulz Moore J. and McLaws M-L. The coroner's role in the prevention of elder abuse: a study of Australian Coroner's Court cases involving pressure ulcers in elders Journal of Law and Medicine 2018 26 494 https://pubmed.ncbi.nlm.nih.gov/30574733/

Sharp CA, Schulz Moore J. and McLaws M-L. Two-Hourly Repositioning for Prevention of pressure ulcers in the Elderly: Patient Safety or Elder Abuse? Journal of Bioethical Inquiry Published online 22 Jan 2019 https://doi.10.1007/s11673-018-9892-3.

Sharp CA and Campbell J. Reducing skin tears, workload, and costs in the frail aged: replacing showers with bath cloths. AJMS Vol 13 No 2 1$^{st}$ February 2022 https://doi.org/10.3126/ajms.v13i2.40548

Sharp CA and Campbell J. Preventing Pressure Ulcers in aged care by auditing, and changing, work practices. AJMS Vol 13 No 4 1$^{st}$ April 2022. https://doi.org/10.3126/ajms.v13i4.41855 (This research features the Nodec A alternating pressure air mattress)

Sharp CA Do Clinical Practice Guidelines for the Prevention of Pressure Ulcers really prevent Pressure Ulcers? An analysis of the Guidelines. AJMS Vol 13 No 5 1$^{st}$ June 2022. https://DOI:10.3126/ajms.v13i6.43030

**These are all available on Google Scholar at no cost and may help families when their ageing relatives are in hospital or in residential aged care.**